The Supe
Cookbook for Beginners

Quick and Tasty Main and Side Dishes Recipes to Boost Your Diet and Improve Your Skills

Carey Sims

Table of Contents

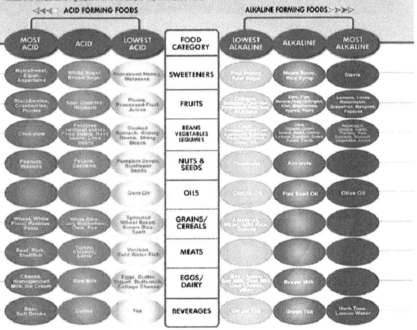

ALKALINE / ACID FOOD CHART

Most high-protein foods (such as meat, fish, poultry and eggs), nearly all carbohydrates (including grains, breads and pastas) and fats are "acid-forming." And most fruits and vegetables are "alkaline-forming." Although citrus fruits, such as oranges and grapefruit, contain organic acids and may have an acid taste, they are not acid-forming when metabolized, leaving no acidic residue. Similarly, Free Form Amino Acids are not acid-forming, but instead offer unique buffering capabilities to the body to help offset acidic wastes.

ACID FORMING FOODS				ALKALINE FORMING FOODS		
MOST ACID	ACID	LOWEST ACID	FOOD CATEGORY	LOWEST ALKALINE	ALKALINE	MOST ALKALINE
NutraSweet, Equal, Aspartame	White Sugar, Brown Sugar	Processed Honey, Molasses	SWEETENERS	Raw Honey, Raw Sugar	Maple Syrup, Rice Syrup	Stevia
Blackberries, Cranberries, Prunes	Sour Cherries, Rhubarb	Plums, Processed Fruit Juices	FRUITS	Oranges, Bananas, Cherries, Pineapple, Peaches, Avocado	Dates, Figs, Melons, Grapes, Kiwi, Blueberries, Apples, Pears	Lemons, Limes, Watermelon, Grapefruit, Mangoes, Papaya
Chocolate	Potatoes (without skins), Pinto Beans, Navy Beans, Lima Beans	Cooked Spinach, Kidney Beans, String Beans	BEANS VEGETABLES LEGUMES	Carrots, Tomatoes, Fresh Corn, Mushrooms, Cabbage, Peas	Okra, Squash, Green Beans, Beets, Celery, Lettuce, Zucchini, Sweet Potato, Carob	Asparagus, Onions, Garlic, Parsley, Raw Spinach, Broccoli, Vegetable Juices
Peanuts, Walnuts	Pecans, Cashews	Pumpkin Seeds, Sunflower Seeds	NUTS & SEEDS	Chestnuts	Almonds	
		Corn Oil	OILS	Canola Oil	Flax Seed Oil	Olive Oil
Wheat, White Flour, Pastries, Pasta	White Rice, Corn, Buckwheat, Oats, Rye	Sprouted Wheat Bread, Brown Rice, Spelt	GRAINS/ CEREALS	Amaranth, Millet, Wild Rice, Quinoa		
Beef, Pork, Shellfish	Turkey, Chicken, Lamb	Venison, Cold Water Fish	MEATS			
Cheese, Homogenized Milk, Ice Cream	Raw Milk	Eggs, Butter, Yogurt, Buttermilk, Cottage Cheese	EGGS/ DAIRY	Soy Cheese, Soy Milk, Goat Milk, Goat Cheese, Whey	Breast Milk	
Beer, Soft Drinks	Coffee	Tea	BEVERAGES	Ginger Tea	Green Tea	Herb Teas, Lemon Water

*The colors used for this chart are not directly relative to the pH scale.

Note that a food's acid or alkaline-forming tendency in the body has nothing to do with the actual pH of the food itself. For example, lemons are very acidic, however the end-products they produce after digestion and assimilation are very alkaline so lemons are alkaline-forming in the body. Likewise, meat will test alkaline before digestion but it leaves very acidic residue in the body so, like nearly all animal products, meat is very acid-forming.

ACID / ALKALINE FOOD COMPARISON CHART

◁◁◁ MORE ACIDIC - EAT LESS   NEUTRAL   MORE ALKALINE - EAT MORE ▷▷▷▷

Soft Drinks	Popcorn	Most Purified Water	Fruit Juices	Most Tap Water	Apples	Avocados	pHresh greens®
Energy Drink	Cream Cheese	Distilled Water	Most Grains	Most Spring Water	Almonds	Green Tea	Spinach
Carbonated Drinks	Buttermilk	Coffee	Eggs	River Water	Tomatoes	Lettuce	Broccoli
	Pastries	Chocolate	Fish		Grapefruit	Celery	Artichoke
	Pasta	Sweetened Fruit Juice	Tea		Corn	Peas	Brussel Sprouts
	Cheese	Pistachios	Soy Milk		Mushrooms	Sweet Potatoes	Cabbage
	Pork	White Bread	Coconut		Turnip	Egg Plant	Cauliflower
	Beef	Peanuts	Lima Beans		Olives	Green Beans	Carrots
	Beer, Wine	Nuts	Plums		Peaches	Beets	Cucumbers
	Black Tea	Wheat	Brown Rice		Bell Pepper	Blueberries	Lemons
	Pickles		Cocoa		Radish	Pears	Limes
	Roasted Nuts		Oats		Pineapple	Grapes	Seaweed
	Vinegar		Oysters		Cherries	Kiwi	Asparagus
	Sweet & Low		Salmon		Wild Rice	Melons	Kale
*Processed &	Equal, Nutra Sweet				Apricot	Tangerines	Radish
Refined Food					Strawberries	Figs	Collard Greens
					Bananas	Dates	Onion
						Mangoes	*Raw / Uncooked
						Papayas	

Note that a food's acid or alkaline-forming tendency in the body has nothing to do with the actual pH of the food itself. For example, lemons are very acidic, however the end-products they produce after digestion and assimilation are very alkaline so lemons are alkaline-forming in the body. Likewise, meat will test alkaline before diges tion but it leaves very acidic residue in the body so, like nearly all animal products, meat is very acid-forming.

*Eat less processed and refined foods and more raw and uncooked greens and fruits.

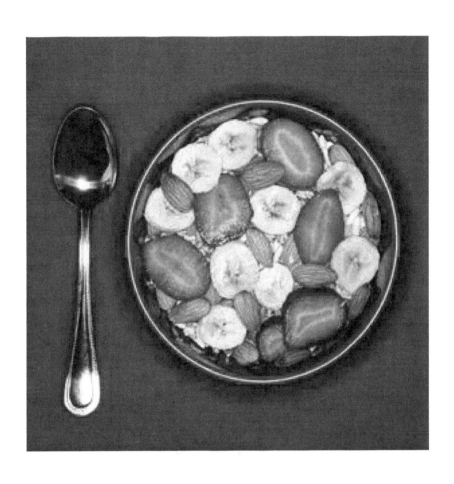

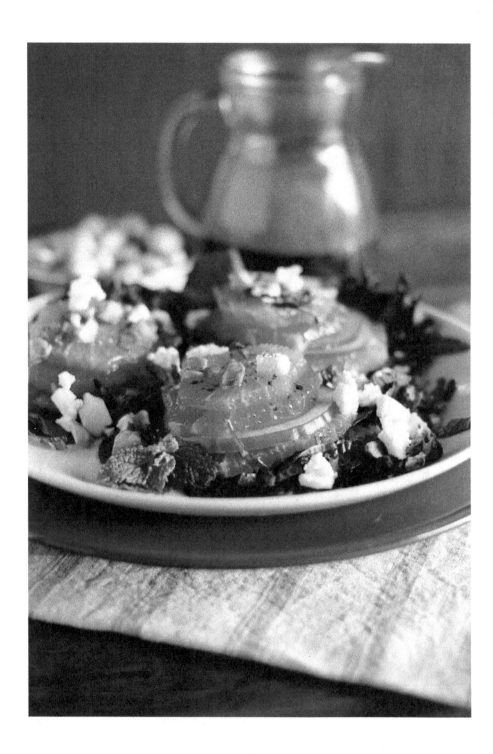

SPICED CAULIFLOWER

Serves: 4

Prep Time: 10 Minutes

Cook Time: 30 Minutes

Total Time: 40 Minutes

INGREDIENTS

- 1 head cauliflower

- 2 tablespoons olive oil

- 1 tsp smoked paprika

- ¼ tsp cumin

- ¼ tsp coriander

- ¼ tsp salt

- ¼ tsp black pepper

DIRECTIONS

1. In a bowl toss the cauliflower with olive oil, paprika, cumin, coriander, salt and pepper

2. Spread the cauliflower on a baking sheet

3. Bake for 20 minutes at 400 F

4. When ready remove from the oven and serve

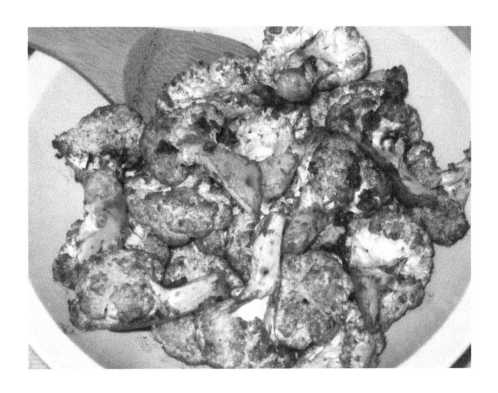

ROASTED BUTTERNUT SQUASH

Serves: *1*

Prep Time: *10* Minutes

Cook Time: *35* Minutes

Total Time: *45* Minutes

INGREDIENTS

- 1 butternut squash

- 2 shallots

- 2 tablespoons olive oil

- 1 tsp rosemary

- ½ tsp salt

- ¼ tsp black pepper

DIRECTIONS

1. In a bowl combine all ingredients together

2. Add the butternut squash in the mixture and let it marinate for 10-15 minutes

3. Bake for 20 minutes at 425 F

4. When ready remove from the oven and serve

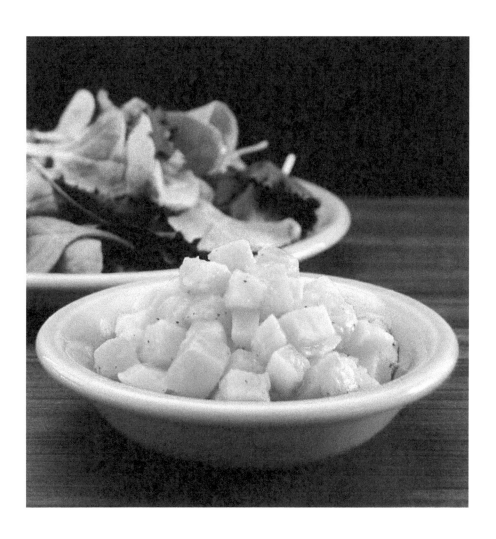

FRIED CHICKEN

Serves: 4

Prep Time: 10 Minutes

Cook Time: 20 Minutes

Total Time: 30 Minutes

INGREDIENTS

- 2 chicken breasts
- ½ cup almond flour
- 1 tsp salt
- 1 tsp black pepper
- 2 eggs
- 1 cup bread crumbs
- ½ cup parmesan cheese

DIRECTIONS

1. In a bowl combine flour, salt and pepper

2. In another bowl beat eggs and add to the flour mixture

3. Cut chicken breasts into thin slices and dip into the flour mixture

4. In another bowl combine bread crumbs and parmesan cheese

5. Take the chicken slices and dip into bread crumbs mixture

6. Place the chicken in frying pan and cook until golden brown

7. When ready remove from the pan and serve

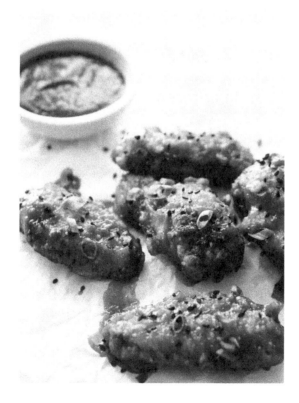

ROASTED CHICKEN

Serves: 4-6

Prep Time: 10   Minutes

Cook Time: 40   Minutes

Total Time: 50   Minutes

INGREDIENTS

-         1 whole chicken

-         1 celery

-         1 onion

-         4 cloves garlic

-         1 sprig of rosemary

-         1 bay leaf

-         1 tablespoon olive oil

-         1 tsp salt

-         1 tsp black pepper

DIRECTIONS

1. In a pot heat olive oil and sauté onion, garlic and celery

2. Add chicken, rosemary, bay leaf, salt, black pepper and cook for 4-5 minutes

3. Remove from the pot and transfer to the oven

4. Bake for 30-35 minutes at 325 F

5. When ready remove from the oven and serve

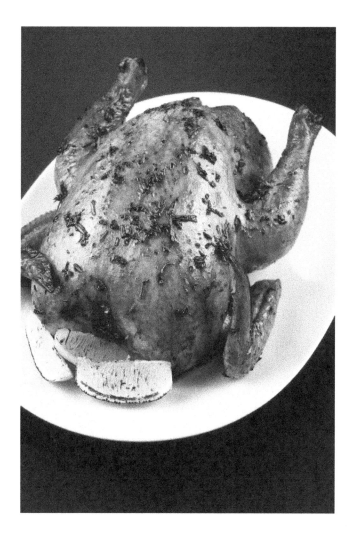

GLAZED SALMON

Serves: *1*

Prep Time: *10* Minutes

Cook Time: *30* Minutes

Total Time: *40* Minutes

INGREDIENTS

- 1 salmon

- ¼ cup brown sugar

- 1 tablespoon lemon zest

- 1 tsp salt

- 1 tsp black pepper

DIRECTIONS

1. In a bowl combine sugar, lemon zest, salt and pepper

2. Spread the mixture over the salmon and rub with the mixture

3. Bake at 350 F for 20-25 minutes

4. When ready remove from the oven and serve

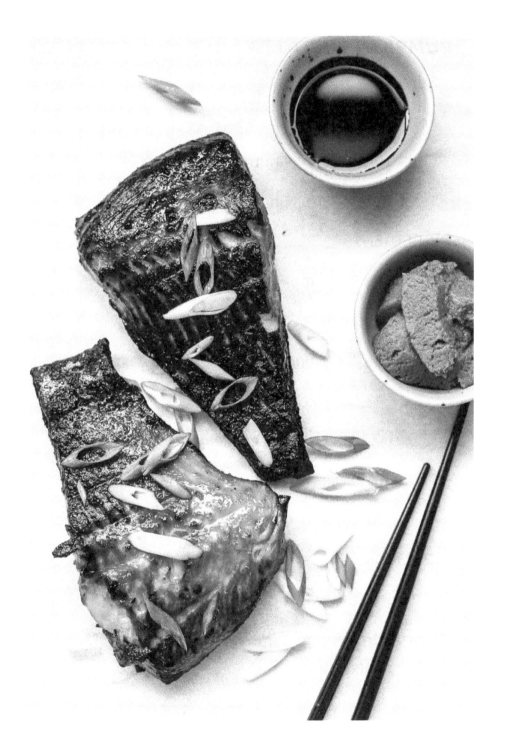

PUMPKIN FRITATTA

Serves: 2

Prep Time: 10 Minutes

Cook Time: 20 Minutes

Total Time: 30 Minutes

INGREDIENTS

- ½ lb. pumpkin puree

- 1 tablespoon olive oil

- ½ red onion

- ¼ tsp salt

- 2 oz. cheddar cheese

- 1 garlic clove

- ¼ tsp dill

DIRECTIONS

1. In a bowl whisk eggs with salt and cheese

2. In a frying pan heat olive oil and pour egg mixture

3. Add remaining ingredients and mix well

4. Serve when ready

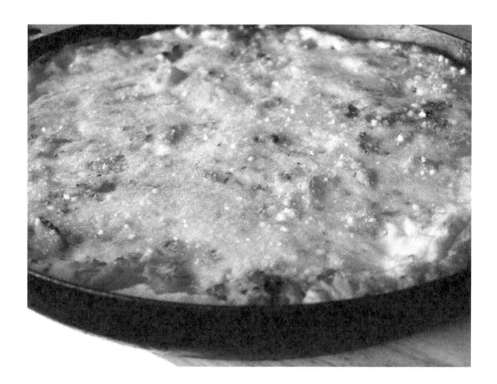

SPINACH FRITATTA

Serves: *2*

Prep Time: *10*   Minutes

Cook Time: *20*   Minutes

Total Time: *30*   Minutes

INGREDIENTS

- ½ lb. spinach

- 1 tablespoon olive oil

- ½ red onion

- ¼ tsp salt

- 2 oz. cheddar cheese

- 1 garlic clove

- ¼ tsp dill

DIRECTIONS

1. In a bowl whisk eggs with salt and cheese

2. In a frying pan heat olive oil and pour egg mixture

3. Add remaining ingredients and mix well

4. Serve when ready

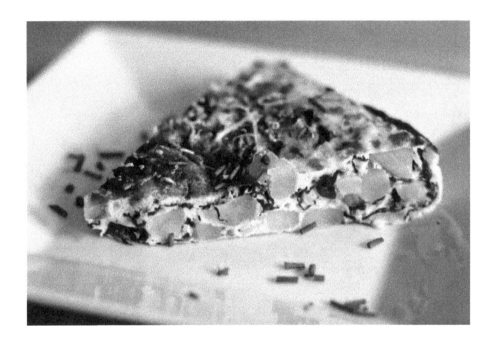

BROCCOLI FRITATTA

Serves: 2

Prep Time: 10   Minutes

Cook Time: 20   Minutes

Total Time: 30   Minutes

INGREDIENTS

-          1 cup broccoli

-          1 tablespoon olive oil

-          ½ red onion

-          ¼ tsp salt

-          2 oz. cheddar cheese

-          1 garlic clove

-          ¼ tsp dill

DIRECTIONS

1. In a skillet sauté broccoli until tender

2. In a bowl whisk eggs with salt and cheese

3. In a frying pan heat olive oil and pour egg mixture

4. Add remaining ingredients and mix well

5. When ready serve with sautéed broccoli

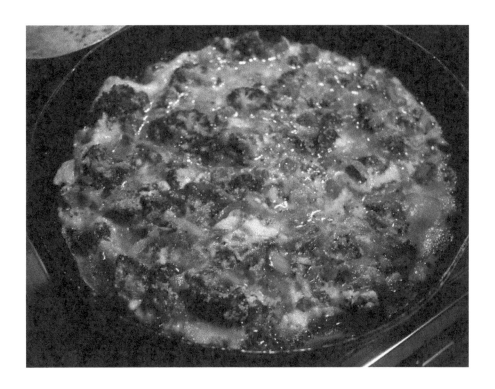

SALMON WITH HERB SAUCE

Serves: *2*

Prep Time: *10* Minutes

Cook Time: *35* Minutes

Total Time: *45* Minutes

INGREDIENTS

- 2 salmon fillets

- 2 tablespoons butter

- 1 tablespoon flour

- 1 tsp tarragon

- 5-6 sage leaves

- 1 tablespoon parsley

DIRECTIONS

1. In a dish combine all ingredients together except the salmon fillets

2. Spread the mixture over the salmon fillet and rub the fish with it

3. Place the salmon in the oven at 325 F for 30-35 minutes

4. When ready remove from the oven and serve

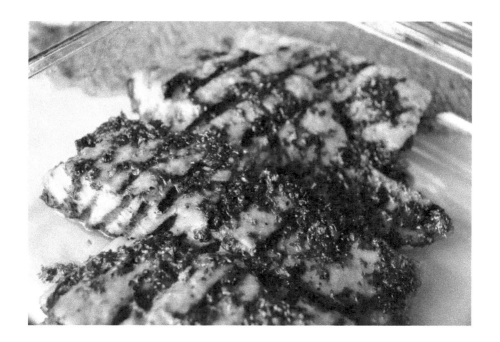

GLAZED PORK CHOPS

Serves: *2*

Prep Time: *10* Minutes

Cook Time: *20* Minutes

Total Time: *30* Minutes

INGREDIENTS

- ½ cup dark rum

- ¼ cup maple syrup

- ¼ cup olive oil

- 2 pork chops

- marinade

DIRECTIONS

1. In a bowl prepare the marinade for the pork chops and set aside

2. Add the pork chops to marinade, refrigerate for 50-60 minutes

3. Place the rum, maple syrup and olive oil in a saucepan and bring to a boil

4. Place the pork chops in a skillet and cook on low heat

5. Pour glaze from the saucepan over the pork chops and cook until pork chops are cooked

6. When ready transfer to a plate and serve

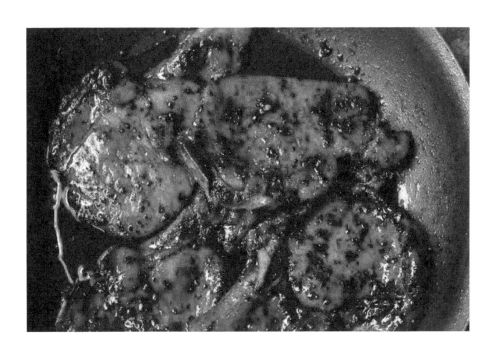

CACIO E PEPE PIZZA

Serves: *6-8*

Prep Time: *10*   Minutes

Cook Time: *15*   Minutes

Total Time: *25*   Minutes

INGREDIENTS

- 1 pizza crust

- ½ cup tomato sauce

- 1 tablespoon olive oil

- 2 oz. parmesan cheese

- 1 tsp black peppercorns

- 4-5 tablespoons ricotta cheese

DIRECTIONS

1. Spread tomato sauce on the pizza crust

2. Place all the toppings on the pizza crust

3. Bake the pizza at 425 F for 12-15 minutes

4. When ready remove pizza from the oven and serve

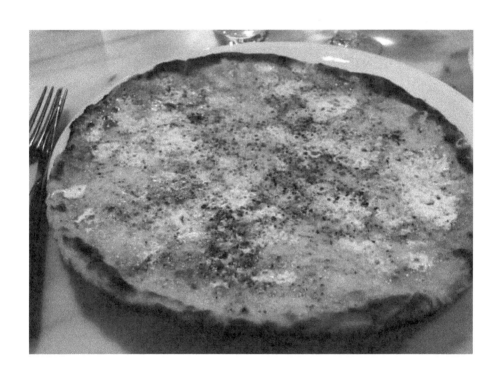

FENNEL PIZZA

Serves: *6-8*

Prep Time: *10*   Minutes

Cook Time: *15*   Minutes

Total Time: *25*   Minutes

INGREDIENTS

- 1 pizza crust
- 1 garlic clove
- 1 tablespoon olive oil
- 1 can cherry tomatoes
- 4-5 pork sausages
- 1 tsp fennel seeds
- 2-3 basil leaves

DIRECTIONS

1. Spread tomato sauce on the pizza crust
2. Place all the toppings on the pizza crust
3. Bake the pizza at 425 F for 12-15 minutes

4. When ready remove pizza from the oven and serve

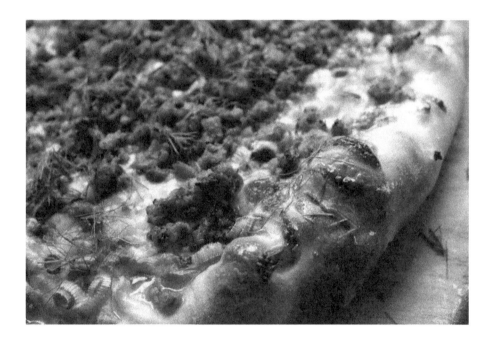

ARTICHOKE PIZZA

Serves: 6-8

Prep Time: 10   Minutes

Cook Time: 15   Minutes

Total Time: 25   Minutes

INGREDIENTS

-        1 pizza crust

-        1 garlic clove

-        1 can tomatoes

-        1 cup mozzarella

-        1 cup olives

-        1 tablespoon capers

-        2-3 artichoke hearts

DIRECTIONS

1. Spread tomato sauce on the pizza crust

2. Place all the toppings on the pizza crust

3. Bake the pizza at 425 F for 12-15 minutes

4. When ready remove pizza from the oven and serve

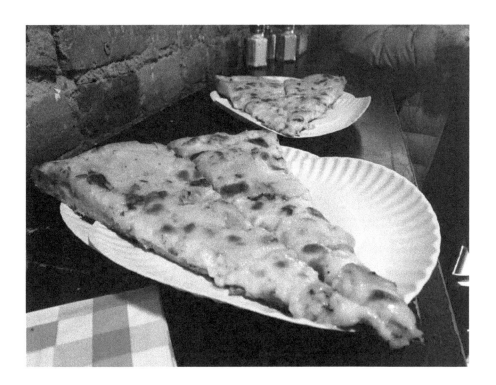

VEGGIES PIZZA

Serves: *1*

Prep Time: *10*   Minutes

Cook Time: *15*   Minutes

Total Time: *25*   Minutes

INGREDIENTS

- ½ cup zucchini

- ½ cup mushrooms

- ¼ cup black olives

- 1 pizza dough

- ½ cup tomato sauce

- ¼ cup parmesan cheese

- 1 cup mozzarella cheese

- Olive oil

DIRECTIONS

1. In a bowl combine all vegetables and drizzle olive oil and salt over vegetables

2. On a pizza dough spread tomato sauce, vegetables and top with mozzarella and parmesan cheese

3. Bake at 400 F for 12-15 minutes

4. When ready remove from the oven and serve

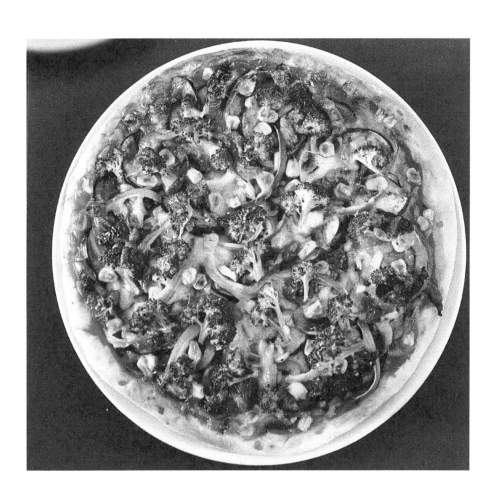

ROASTED BEET

Serves: *3-4*

Prep Time: *10*   Minutes

Cook Time: *20*   Minutes

Total Time: *30*   Minutes

INGREDIENTS

-        2 lb. beet

-        2 tablespoons olive oil

-        1 tsp curry powder

-        1 tsp salt

DIRECTIONS

1. Preheat the oven to 400 F

2. Cut everything in half lengthwise

3. Toss everything with olive oil and place onto a prepared baking sheet

4. Roast for 18-20 minutes at 400 F or until golden brown

5. When ready remove from the oven and serve

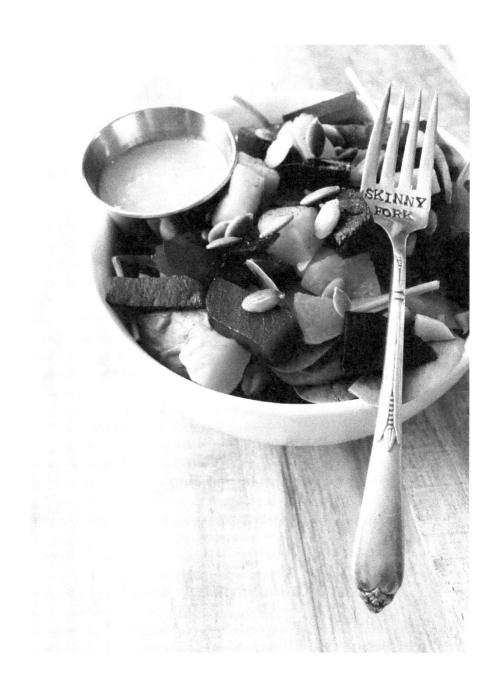

ROASTED SQUASH

Serves: 3-4

Prep Time: 10 Minutes

Cook Time: 20 Minutes

Total Time: 30 Minutes

INGREDIENTS

- 2 delicata squashes

- 2 tablespoons olive oil

- 1 tsp curry powder

- 1 tsp salt

DIRECTIONS

1. Preheat the oven to 400 F

2. Cut everything in half lengthwise

3. Toss everything with olive oil and place onto a prepared baking sheet

4. Roast for 18-20 minutes at 400 F or until golden brown

5. When ready remove from the oven and serve

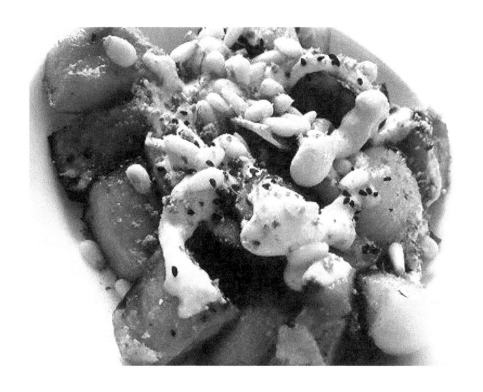

BEEF POT ROAST

Serves: 3

Prep Time: 20 minutes

Cook Time: 60 minutes

Total Time: 80 minutes

INGREDIENTS

- 2 to 4 lbs chuck roast

- heel of round or round bone roast

DIRECTIONS

1. Trim off excess fat

2. Place a tablespoon of oil in a large skillet and heat to medium

3. Roll pot roast in flour and brown on all sides in hot skillet

4. After meat gets a brown color reduce heat to low

5. Season with pepper and herbs and add ½ cup of water

6. Cook slowly for 1 ½ hours or until it looks ready

**You can use vegetables suck as carrots, onions, cabbage

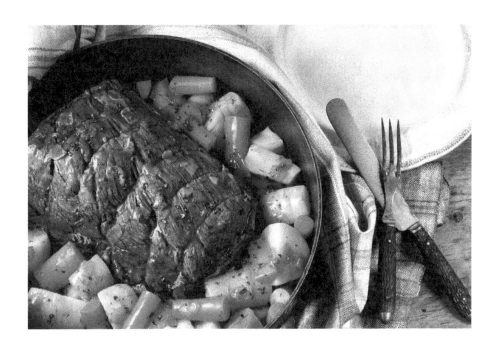

ZUCCHINI SOUP

Serves: *4*

Prep Time: *10* Minutes

Cook Time: *20* Minutes

Total Time: *30* Minutes

INGREDIENTS

- 1 tablespoon olive oil

- 1 lb. zucchini

- ¼ red onion

- ½ cup all-purpose flour

- ¼ tsp salt

- ¼ tsp pepper

- 1 can vegetable broth

- 1 cup heavy cream

DIRECTIONS

1. In a saucepan heat olive oil and sauté zucchini until tender

2. Add remaining ingredients to the saucepan and bring to a boil

3. When all the vegetables are tender transfer to a blender and blend until smooth

4. Pour soup into bowls, garnish with parsley and serve

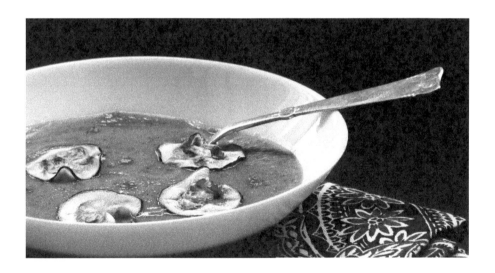

MEAT LOAF

Serves: *1*

Prep Time: *20* minutes

Cook Time: *20* minutes

Total Time: *40* minutes

INGREDIENTS

-        1 lbs lean ground beef

-        1 cup 2% milk

-        1 egg

-        ½ pound lean ground pork 4 slices soft bread

-        ¼ cup onion

-        ¼ teaspoon peeper

-        ¼ teaspoon mustard

-        ¼ teaspoon garlic powder

-        1 tablespoon chopped parsley

-        ½ teaspoon ground sage

DIRECTIONS

1. Heat oven at 350 degrees

2. Mix elements in a bowl

3. Place mixture in a shallow baking dish

4. Bake ½ hours or until done (At the end loaf should be crispy brown)

5. Double recipe can be used for sandwiches for added variety

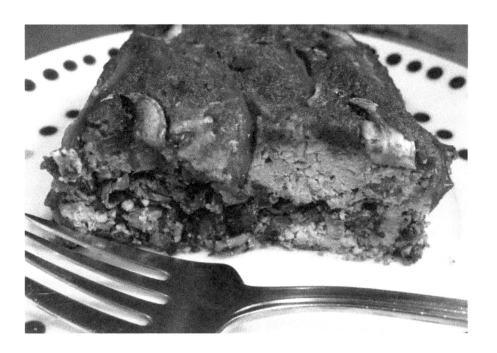

FLANK STEAK WITH HERB SAUCE

Serves: *4*

Prep Time: *20*   minutes

Cook Time: *110*   minutes

Total Time: *130*   minutes

INGREDIENTS

- 2 tablespoons butter

- 2 tablespoons finely chopped onion

- 1 tablespoon cornstarch

- ¼ teaspoon garlic powder

- 1 clove garlic

- ½ teaspoon marjoram

- ½ teaspoon ground oregano

- ¾ cup water

- 2 teaspoons lemon juice

- 2 tablespoons chopped parsley

DIRECTIONS

1. Melt butter in saucepan over low heat

2. Blend in cornstarch

3. Add chopped onions/garlic

4. Remove from heat and stir in herbs

5. Add lemon juice and water

6. Get back to medium heat, season with pepper and then reduce heat

7. Slice broiled frank steak on angle across grain

8. Serve topped with sauce

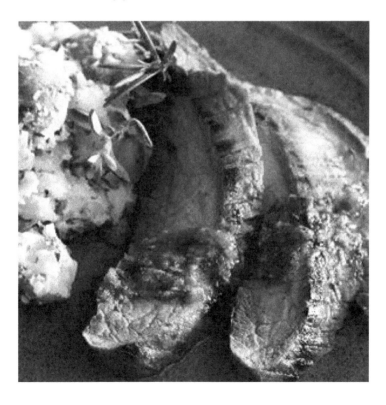

HERB BEEF PATTIES

Serves: *4*

Prep Time: *20*   minutes

Cook Time: *20*   minutes

Total Time: *40*   minutes

INGREDIENTS

-     1 lbs lean ground beef

-     1 tablespoon lemon juice

-     ¼ teaspoon ground thyme

-     ¼ teaspoon rosemary

-     1 teaspoon parsley

DIRECTIONS

1. Mix all ingredients

2. Shape them into four patties

3. Cook on indoor/outdoor grill until meat is brown

4. Spoon out fat as meat cooks

5. Garnish with green pepper and lemon in
   center of ring

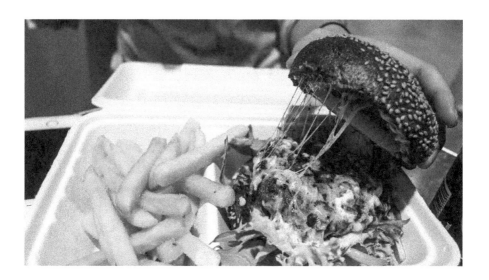

SPAGHETTI WITH MEAT SAUCE

Serves: 8

Prep Time: 20   minutes

Cook Time: 40   minutes

Total Time: 60   minutes

INGREDIENTS

-        1 ½ pounds lean ground beef

-        2 cloves garlic

-        ½ cup onion

-        2 12 oz cans of tomatoes, no added salt

-        2 tablespoons parsley

-        1 cup tomato liquid

-        2 teaspoons oregano leaves

-        ¼ teaspoon black pepper

-        ½ teaspoon thyme

-        1 bay leaf

-        2 tablespoons water

-        2 tablespoons cornstarch

-        10 oz. spaghetti

DIRECTIONS

1. Heat the skillet to medium

2. Cook beef until brown

3. Drain excess fat and reduce heat

4. Add onions and garlic

5. Drain liquid from canned tomatoes and dice the canned tomatoes to the meat

6. Add sugar, parsley and remaining ingredients

7. Add cornstarch and water and 1 tablespoon of olive oil to spaghetti after cooking

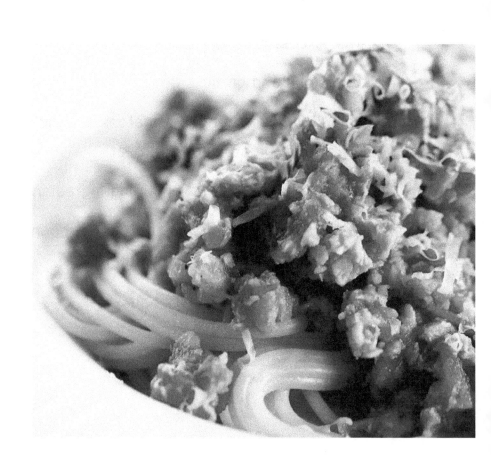

BARBEQUED BEEFIES

Serves: *2*

Prep Time: *15* minutes

Cook Time: *45* minutes

Total Time: *60* minutes

INGREDIENTS

-          1 meat loaf recipe

-          ½ medium onion

-          barbecue sauce

DIRECTIONS

1. Shape mixture into 8 individual loaves

2. Place in baking dish about one inch apart

3. Top each loaf with 1-2 onion slices

4. Pour barbecue sauce over the loaves

5. Bake in 350 degrees for 45 minutes

6. Baste with sauce every 15 minutes while baking

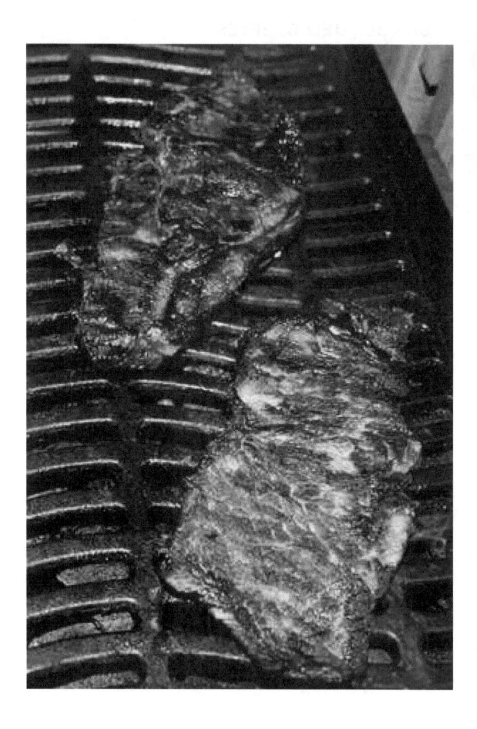

TOMATO MEAT SAUCE

Serves: *4*

Prep Time: *20*   minutes

Cook Time: *60*   minutes

Total Time: *80*   minutes

INGREDIENTS

-          1 tablespoon vegetable oil

-          ½ cup onion

-          ¼ chopped pepper

-          2 lbs lean ground beef

-          ¼ teaspoon pepper

-          ¼ teaspoon chili powder

-          3 ½ cups canned tomatoes

DIRECTIONS

1. Heat oil, onions and green peppers

2. Cook at medium heat until onions are ready

3. Add ground beef, breaking into small pieces

4. Cook until meat gets a brown color and then reduce heat

5. Blend in canned tomatoes

6. Cover for one hour

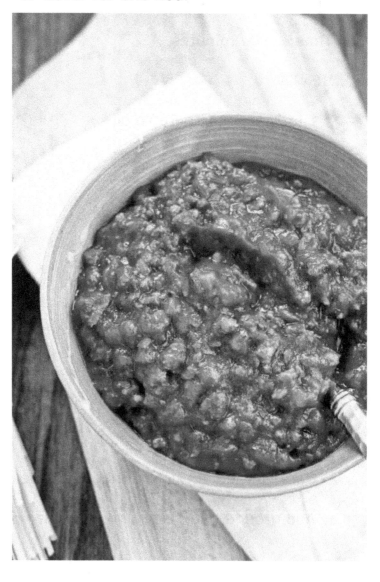

CHICKEN ITALIANO

Serves: *4*

Prep Time: *20*   minutes

Cook Time: *90*   minutes

Total Time: *110*   minutes

INGREDIENTS

-        8 boneless chicken breasts

-        3 tablespoons olive oil

-        ¾ crushed no-salt cracker crumbs

-        1 teaspoon oregano leaves

-        1 teaspoon paprika

-        ¼ teaspoon garlic powder

-        ¼ teaspoon black pepper

DIRECTIONS

1. Add olive oil over chicken

2. Combine all the ingredients

3. Roll chicken pieces in the mixture

4. Bake at 350 degrees for 1hour and 30 minutes

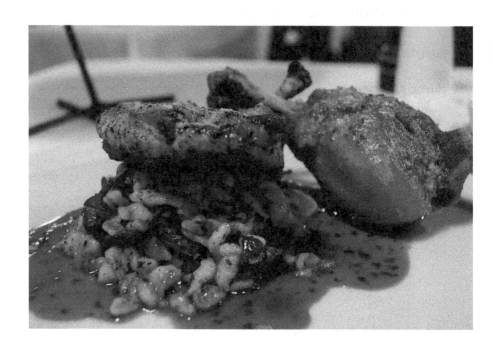

GREEN PESTO PASTA

Serves: *2*

Prep Time: *5*   Minutes

Cook Time: *15* Minutes

Total Time: *20* Minutes

INGREDIENTS

- 4 oz. spaghetti

- 2 cups basil leaves

- 2 garlic cloves

- ¼ cup olive oil

- 2 tablespoons parmesan cheese

- ½ tsp black pepper

DIRECTIONS

1. Bring water to a boil and add pasta

2. In a blend add parmesan cheese, basil leaves, garlic and blend

3. Add olive oil, pepper and blend again

4. Pour pesto onto pasta and serve when ready

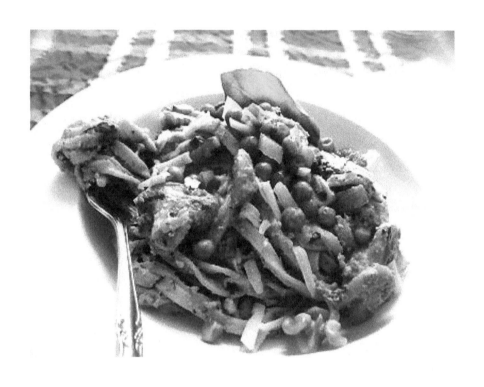

BROCCOLI CRUSTLESS QUICHE

Serves: 6

Prep Time: 10   Minutes

Cook Time: 50   Minutes

Total Time: 60   Minutes

INGREDIENTS

- 1 onion

- 3 oz. raising flour

- 1 lb. broccoli florets

- 1 red capsicum

- 1/3 lb. cheddar cheese

- 1.5 oz. parmesan cheese

- 3 eggs

- 1 lb. milk

DIRECTIONS

1. Preheat oven to 300 F

2. In a dish add veggies, onions and grated cheese

3. In a bowl mix flour, eggs and whisk to combine, add milk and whisk to combine

4. Pour mixture into dish and bake for 40 minutes or until golden brown

5. Remove, let it cool and serve

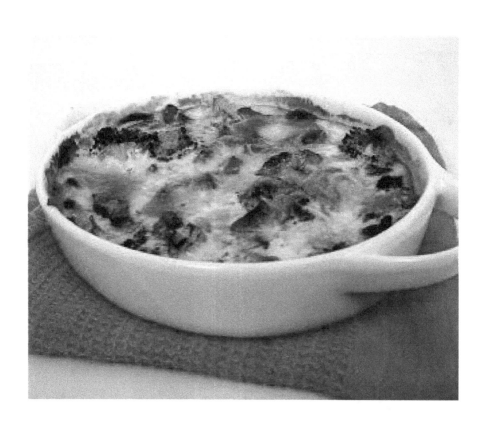

CHEESE AND PESTO TART

Serves: *2*

Prep Time: *10* Minutes

Cook Time: *30* Minutes

Total Time: *40* Minutes

INGREDIENTS

-          1 sheet puff pastry

-          1 handful cherry tomatoes

-          1 handful Kalamata olive

-          2 tablespoon kale and basil pesto

-          2,5 oz. cheddar cheese

-          1 tablespoon pine nuts

DIRECTIONS

1. Preheat oven at 300 F and line a baking sheet

2. Place pastry sheet on baking tray, fork the pastry all over the center of the pastry

3. Spread the pesto over the center of the tart, top with tomatoes, olives and top with grated cheese, top with pine nuts

4. Bake for 20 minutes, remove and serve

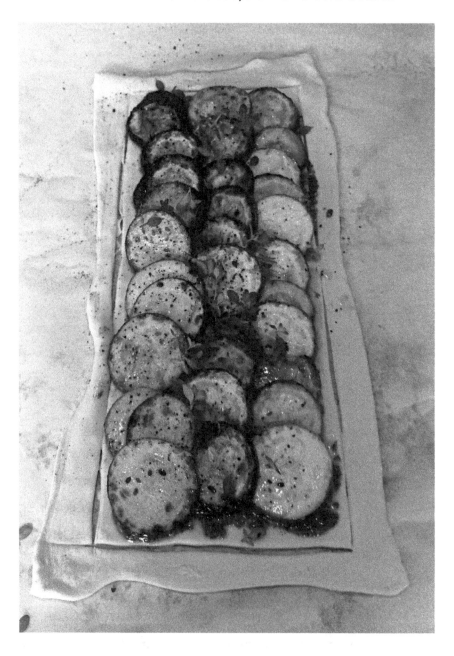

PORK ASIAN SALAD

Serves: *2*

Prep Time: *10* Minutes

Cook Time: *10* Minutes

Total Time: *20* Minutes

INGREDIENTS

- 1 lb. shredded pork

- ½ red cabbage

- 3 carrots

- 4 onions

- 1 red chili

- ½ bunch coriander

DRESSING

- 3 tablespoons hoisin sauce

- 1 tablespoon sesame oil

DIRECTIONS

1. In a bowl mix all salad ingredients

2. In a jar mix all dressing ingredients

3. Pour dressing over salad and serve

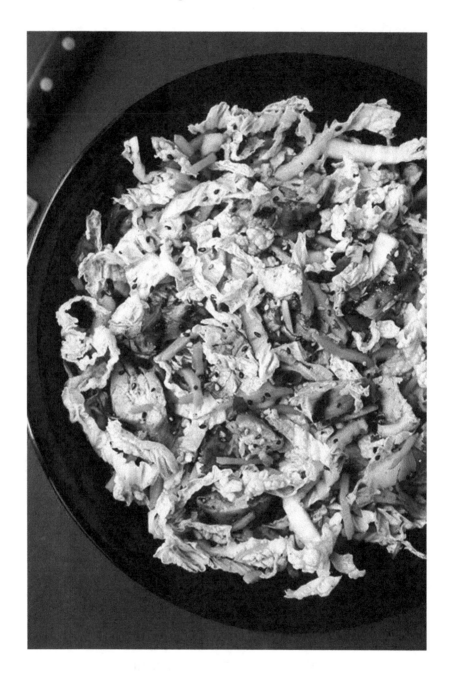

CHILI PRAWN FRY

Serves: *4*

Prep Time: *10*   Minutes

Cook Time: *20*   Minutes

Total Time: *30*   Minutes

INGREDIENTS

-         2 carrots

-         ¼ lb. snow peas

-         1 tsp olive oil

-         1 garlic clove

-         1 green chili

-         1 tablespoon soy sauce

-         1 tablespoon wine

-         1 tsp sesame oil

-         ½ lb. prawns

-          noodles

DIRECTIONS

1. In a wok add oil, garlic, chili, veggies and cook over medium heat for 2-3 minutes

2. In a pot boil noodles

3. Add sesame oil, soy sauce into the wok and cook for 2-3 minutes

4. Add the prawns and fry for 2-3 minutes, serve with noodles

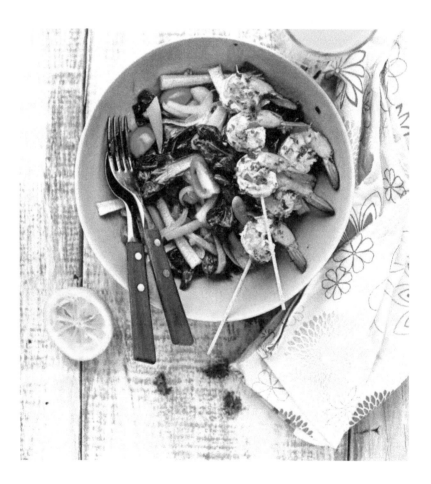

ZUCCHINI LASAGNE

Serves: *4*

Prep Time: *10*   Minutes

Cook Time: *30*   Minutes

Total Time: *40*   Minutes

INGREDIENTS

-         1 tablespoon olive oil

-         1 onion

-         3 garlic cloves

-         1,5 lb. zucchini

-          ½ lb. quark

-         2 oz. cheddar cheese

-         1 oz. pizza cheese

-         3 lasagna sheets

-         1 lb. tomato pasta sauce

DIRECTIONS

1. Preheat oven to 350 F

2. In a frying pan fry onion for 2-3 minutes, add garlic, zucchini, garlic and cook for another 2-3 minutes

3. Stir in 2/3 quark, cheddar cheese and season

4. Heat the tomato sauce and layer up a baking dish, add zucchini mixture, lasagna sheets, tomato sauce and remaining quark

5. Sprinkle the cheddar cheese and pizza cheese

6. Bake for 15-20 minutes or until golden brown

7. Remove and serve

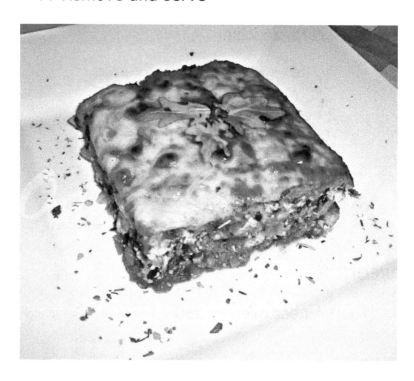

FRIED VEGETABLES

Serves: *2*

Prep Time: *10* Minutes

Cook Time: *15* Minutes

Total Time: *25* Minutes

INGREDIENTS

-      1 cup red bell pepper

-      ¼ cup cucumber

-      ¼ cup zucchini

-      ¼ cup asparagus

-      ¼ cup carrots

-      1 onion

-      2 eggs

-      1 tsp salt

-      1 tsp pepper

-      Seasoning

-      1 tablespoon olive oil

DIRECTIONS

1. In a skillet heat olive oil and sauté onion until soft

2. Chop vegetables into thin slices and pour over onion

3. Whisk eggs with salt and pepper and pour over the vegetables

4. Cook until vegetables are brown

5. When ready remove from heat and serve

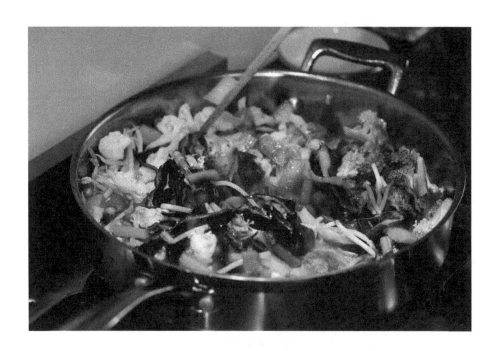

ONION SAUCE

Serves: *4*

Prep Time: *10* Minutes

Cook Time: *55* Minutes

Total Time: *65* Minutes

INGREDIENTS

-        1 onion

-        2 garlic cloves

-        ¼ lb. carrots

-        1 potato

-        1 tablespoon balsamic vinegar

-        ¼ tsp salt

-        ¼ tsp black pepper

-        1 tablespoon olive oil

-        1 cup water

DIRECTIONS

1. Chop all the vegetables and place them in a heated skillet

2. Add remaining ingredients and cook on low heat

3. Allow to simmer for 40-45 minutes or until vegetables are soft

4. Transfer mixture to a blender and blend until smooth

5. When ready remove from the blender and serve

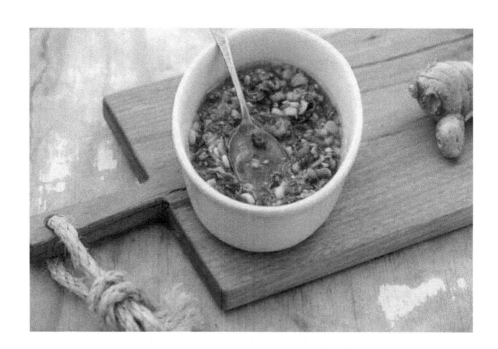

FISH "CAKE"

Serves: *4-6*

Prep Time: *10*   Minutes

Cook Time: *50*   Minutes

Total Time: *60*   Minutes

INGREDIENTS

-        2 tuna tins

-        2 potatoes

-        2 eggs

-        1 handful of gluten free flour

-        1 handful of parsley

-        black pepper

-        1 cup breadcrumbs

DIRECTIONS

1. Preheat the oven to 350 F

2. Boil the potatoes until they are soft

3. Mix the tuna with parsley, black pepper and salt

4. Roll fish into patties and dip into a bowl with flour, then eggs and then breadcrumbs

5. Place the patties on a baking tray

6. Bake at 350 F for 40-45 minutes

7. When ready remove from heat and serve

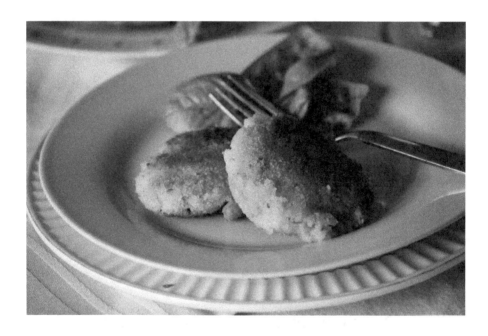

SUSHI HANDROLLS

Serves: *2*

Prep Time: *10* Minutes

Cook Time: *25* Minutes

Total Time: *35* Minutes

INGREDIENTS

- 1 sushi nori packet

- 4 tablespoons mayonnaise

- ½ lb. smoked salmon

- 1 tsp wasabi

- 1 cup cooked sushi rice

- 1 avocado

DIRECTIONS

1. Cut avocado and into thin slices

2. Take a sheet of sushi and spread mayonnaise onto the sheet

3. Add rice, salmon and avocado

4. Roll and dip sushi into wasabi and serve

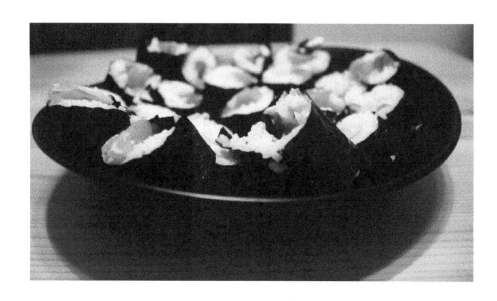

STEAMED VEGETABLES

Serves: 2

Prep Time: 10   Minutes

Cook Time: 10   Minutes

Total Time: 20   Minutes

INGREDIENTS

-        1 carrot

-        2 sweet potato

-        2 parsnips

-        1 zucchini

-         2 broccoli stems

DIRECTIONS

1. Chop vegetables into thin slices

2. Place all the vegetables into a steamer

3. Add enough water and cook on high until vegetables are steamed

4. When ready remove from the steamer and serve

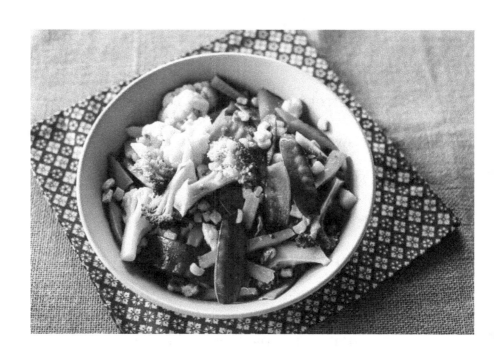

GUACAMOLE

Serves: *2*

Prep Time: *5* Minutes

Cook Time: *5* Minutes

Total Time: *10* Minutes

INGREDIENTS

- 1 avocado

- 1 lime juice

- 1 handful of coriander

- 1 tsp olive oil

- 1 tsp salt

- 1 tsp pepper

DIRECTIONS

1. Place all the ingredients in a blender

2. Blend until smooth and transfer to a bowl

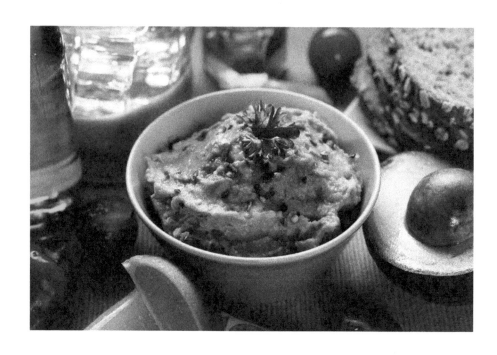

CHICKEN NACHOS

Serves: 4-6

Prep Time: 15   Minutes

Cook Time: 35   Minutes

Total Time: 50   Minutes

INGREDIENTS

-      2 chicken breasts

-       Tortilla chips

-      Fajita seasoning

-      ¼ cup cheddar cheese

-      4-5 mushrooms

-      Guacamole

-      ¼ cup peppers

DIRECTIONS

1. In a pan heat olive oil and add chopped onion, sauté until soft

2. Add chicken, fajita seasoning and remaining vegetables

3. Cook on low heat for 10-12 minutes

4. Place tortilla chips into a baking dish, sprinkle cheese and bake in the oven until cheese has melted

5. Remove from the oven pour sautéed vegetables and chicken over and tortilla chips and serve

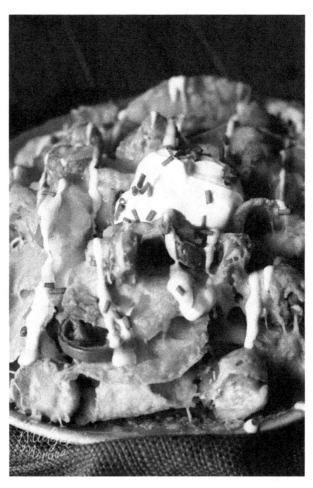

SCRAMBLED EGGS WITH SALMON

Serves: *2*

Prep Time: *10* Minutes

Cook Time: *20* Minutes

Total Time: *30* Minutes

INGREDIENTS

- ½ lb. smoked salmon

- 2 eggs

- 1 avocado

- 1 tsp salt

- 1 tsp pepper

- 1 tps olive oil

DIRECTIONS

1. In a bowl whisk the eggs with salt and pepper

2. In a skillet heat olive oil and pour the egg mixture

3. Add salmon pieces to the mixture and cook for 2-3 minutes per side

4. When ready remove from the skillet, add
   avocado and serve

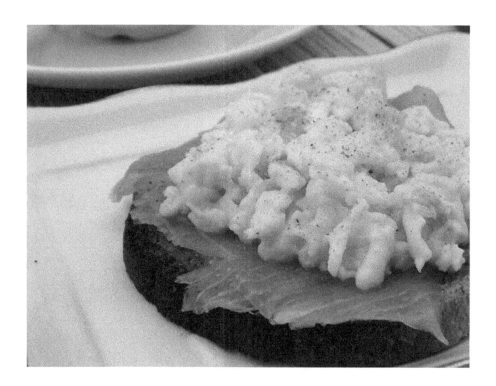

CHICKEN WITH RICE

Serves: *4*

Prep Time: *10*   Minutes

Cook Time: *25*   Minutes

Total Time: *35*   Minutes

INGREDIENTS

-        2 chicken breasts

-        1 cup cooked white rice

-        2 tablespoons mayonnaise

-        1 tablespoon curry powder

-        1 zucchini

-        1 cup broccoli

-        1 tablespoon olive oil

DIRECTIONS

1. Cut chicken breast into small pieces and set aside

2. In a pan heat olive oil and cook the chicken breast for 4-5 minutes

3. In another bowl combine mayonnaise, curry powder and add mixture to the chicken

4. Add remaining ingredients and cook for another 10-12 minutes or until the chicken is ready

5. When ready remove from the pot and serve with white rice

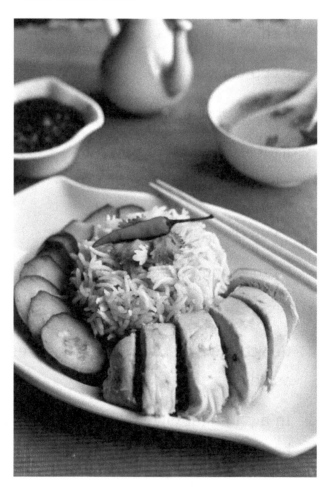

ROASTED VEGETABLES

Serves: *2*

Prep Time: *10* Minutes

Cook Time: *50* Minutes

Total Time: *60* Minutes

INGREDIENTS

-         1 carrot

-         2 sweet potatoes

-         1 butternut squash

-         2 parsnips

-         1 rosemary spring

-         2 bay leaves

DIRECTIONS

1. Chop the vegetables into thin slices

2. Place everything in a prepare baking dish

3. Bake at 350 F for 40-45 minutes or until vegetables are golden brown

4. When ready remove from the oven and serve

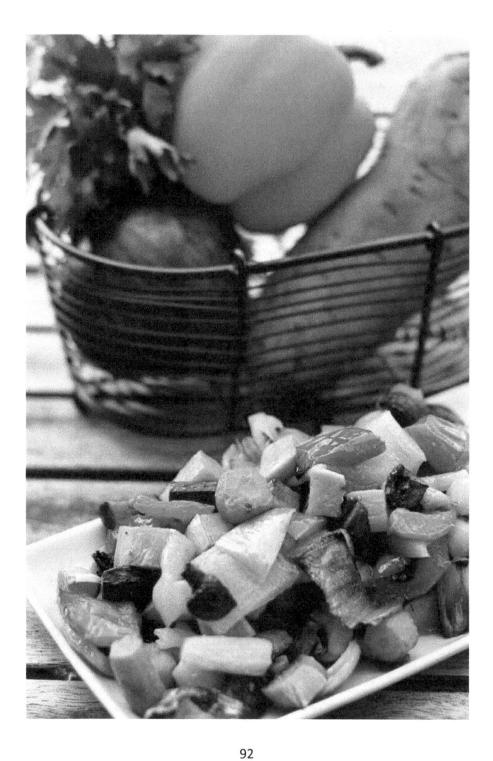

CRANBERRY SALAD

Serves: *2*

Prep Time: *5* Minutes

Cook Time: *5* Minutes

Total Time: *10* Minutes

INGREDIENTS

- 1 can unsweetened pineapple

- 1 package cherry gelatin

- 1 tablespoon lemon juice

- ½ cup artificial sweetener

- 1 cup cranberries

- 1 orange

- 1 cup celery

- ½ cup pecans

DIRECTIONS

1. In a bowl combine all ingredients together and mix well

2. Serve with dressing

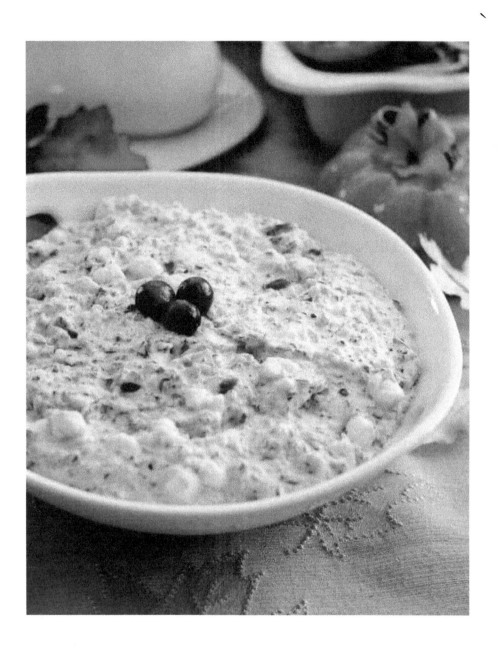

ITALIAN SALAD

Serves: 2

Prep Time: 5   Minutes

Cook Time: 5   Minutes

Total Time: 10   Minutes

INGREDIENTS

-        8 oz. romaine lettuce

-        2 cups radicchio

-        ¼ red onion

-        2 ribs celery

-        1 cup tomatoes

-        1 can chickpeas

-        1 cup salad dressing

DIRECTIONS

1. In a bowl combine all ingredients together and mix well

2.   Serve with dressing

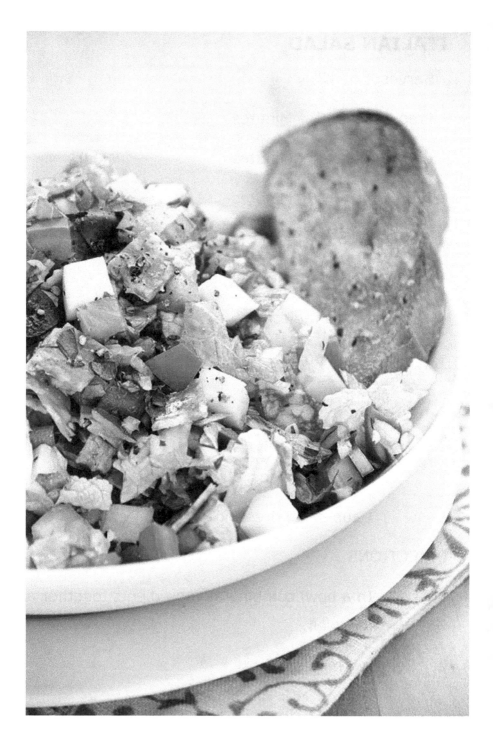

CHICKPEA COLESLAW

Serves: *2*

Prep Time: *5*   Minutes

Cook Time: *5*   Minutes

Total Time: *10*   Minutes

INGREDIENTS

- 2 cans chickpeas

- 2 cups carrots

- 1 cup celery

- ¼ cup green onions

- ¼ cup dill leaves

- ¼ cup olive oil

- 1 cucumber

- 1 cup salad dressing

DIRECTIONS

1. In a bowl combine all ingredients together and mix well

2. Serve with dressing

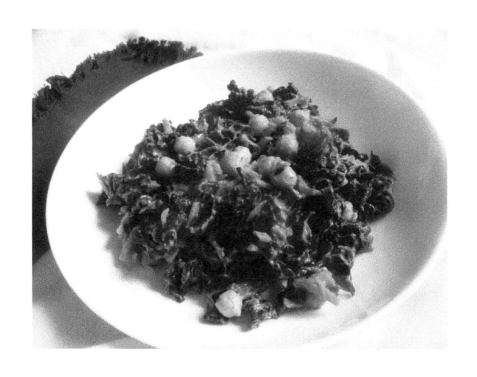

ROMAINE SALAD

Serves: *2*

Prep Time: *5* Minutes

Cook Time: *5* Minutes

Total Time: *10* Minutes

INGREDIENTS

- 1 cup cooked quinoa

- 1 cup sunflower seeds

- 1 tablespoon olive oil

- 1 head romaine lettuce

- 1 cup carrots

- 1 cup cabbage

- ¼ cup radishes

DIRECTIONS

1. In a bowl combine all ingredients together and mix well

2. Serve with dressing

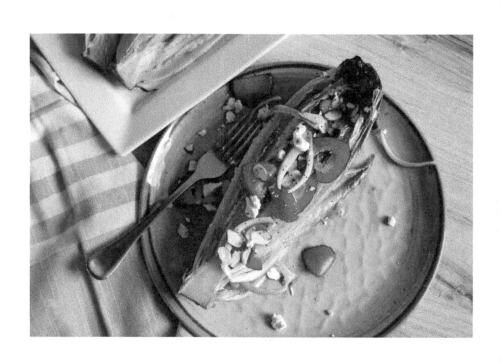

GRAIN SALAD

Serves: *2*

Prep Time: *5* Minutes

Cook Time: *5* Minutes

Total Time: *10* Minutes

INGREDIENTS

- 1 bunch coriander leaves

- 1 bunch mint leaves

- ¼ red onion

- 1 bunch parsley

- 1 cup lentils

- 1 tablespoon pumpkin seeds

- 1 tablespoon pine nuts

DIRECTIONS

1. In a bowl combine all ingredients together and mix well

2. Serve with dressing

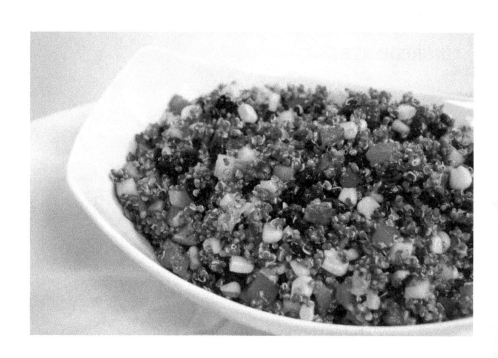

QUINOA SALAD

Serves: *2*

Prep Time: *5*   Minutes

Cook Time: *5*   Minutes

Total Time: *10* Minutes

INGREDIENTS

- 1 cauliflower
- 2 cups cooked quinoa
- 1 can chickpeas
- 1 cup baby spinach
- ¼ cup parsley
- ¼ cup cilantro
- ¼ cup green onion
- ½ cup feta cheese

DIRECTIONS

1. In a bowl combine all ingredients together and mix well

2. Serve with dressing

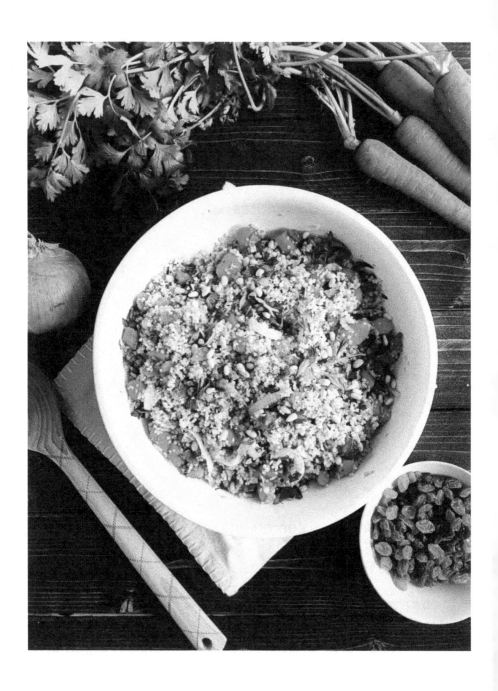

WEDGE SALAD

Serves: 2

Prep Time: 5 Minutes

Cook Time: 5 Minutes

Total Time: 10 Minutes

INGREDIENTS

- 1 head romaine lettuce

- 1 cup tomatoes

- 1 cup cucumber

- 1 cup celery

- ¼ cup olives

- 1 shallot

- 1 cup salad dressing

DIRECTIONS

1. In a bowl combine all ingredients together and mix well

2. Serve with dressing

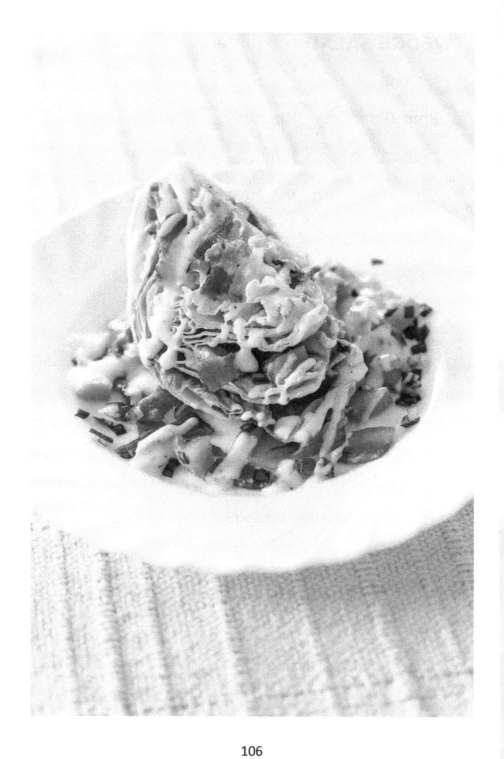

THAI MANGO SALAD

Serves: *2*

Prep Time: *5*   Minutes

Cook Time: *5*   Minutes

Total Time: *10* Minutes

INGREDIENTS

- 1 head leaf lettuce

- 1 red bell pepper

- 2 mangoes

- ¼ green onion

- ¼ cup peanuts

- ¼ cup cilantro

- 1 cup peanut dressing

DIRECTIONS

1. In a bowl combine all ingredients together and mix well

2. Serve with dressing

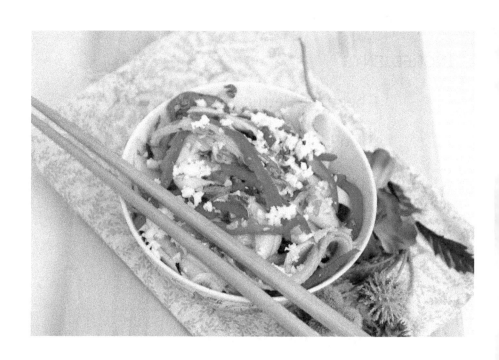

BEEF STEW

Serves: *4*

Prep Time: *15* Minutes

Cook Time: *45* Minutes

Total Time: *60* Minutes

INGREDIENTS

- 2 lb. beef

- 1 tsp salt

- 4 tablespoons olive oil

- 2 red onions

- 2 cloves garlic

- 1 cup white wine

- 2 cups beef broth

- 1 cup water

- 3-4 bay leaves

- ¼ tsp thyme

- 1 lb. potatoes

DIRECTIONS

1. Chop all ingredients in big chunks

2. In a large pot heat olive oil and add ingredients one by one

3. Cook for 5-6 or until slightly brown

4. Add remaining ingredients and cook until tender, 35-45 minutes

5. Season while stirring on low heat

6. When ready remove from heat and serve

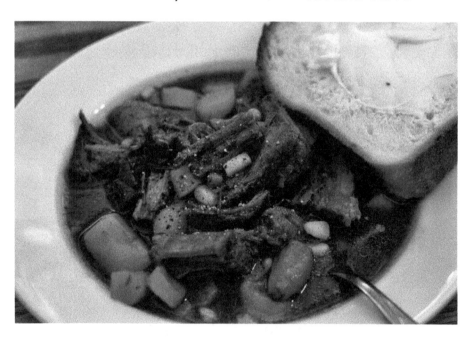

Printed in the USA
CPSIA information can be obtained
at www.ICGtesting.com
LVHW021052150224
771954LV00024B/319